45 Powerful Juice Recipes to Boost Your Immune System:

Strengthen Your Immune System without the Use of Pills or Medical Treatments

By

Joe Correa CSN

COPYRIGHT

This publication is designed to provide accurate and authoritative information in regard to the subject matter covered. It is sold with the understanding that neither the author nor the publisher is engaged in rendering medical advice. If medical advice or assistance is needed, consult with a doctor. This book is considered a guide and should not be used in any way detrimental to your health. Consult with a physician before starting this nutritional plan to make sure it's right for you.

ACKNOWLEDGEMENTS

This book is dedicated to my friends and family that have had mild or serious illnesses so that you may find a solution and make the necessary changes in your life.

45 Powerful Juice Recipes to Boost Your Immune System:

Strengthen Your Immune System without the Use of Pills or Medical Treatments

By

Joe Correa CSN

CONTENTS

ABOUT THE AUTHOR

After years of Research, I honestly believe in the positive effects that proper nutrition can have over the body and mind. My knowledge and experience has helped me live healthier throughout the years and which I have shared with family and friends. The more you know about eating and drinking healthier, the sooner you will want to change your life and eating habits.

Nutrition is a key part in the process of being healthy and living longer so get started today. The first step is the most important and the most significant.

INTRODUCTION

45 Powerful Juice Recipes to Boost Your Immune System: Strengthen Your Immune System without the Use of Pills or Medical Treatments

By Joe Correa CSN

The main reason doctors say people get sick is because of a weak immune system. Having a weak immune system makes it much harder for your body to fight infections, diseases, and any other harmful substances. Exercise and diet are the fastest way to strengthen your immune system. Fruits that are high in vitamin C like strawberries, blueberries, lemon, passion fruit, tangerines, grapefruit, etc.

By including these fruits in your diet on a normal basis you will drastically change your body's capacity to defend itself. The recipes in this book have a variety of ingredients that are vitamin packed and are high in vitamin C which will help you achieve your goal to strengthen your immune system and fight off harmful diseases and infections. Honey and agave syrup are excellent choices when it comes to sweetening your food since they offer a natural source of sugar that your body and quickly absorb. Other potent ingredients we have included are: oats, beetroot, lactose free milk, cereals, peanuts, raisins, pecans, sesame, and linseed, just to name a few.

Make the decision to help your body by giving it what it needs to defend itself. When it comes to getting healthy and staying healthy there's only one choice, eating right!

45 POWERFUL JUICE RECIPES TO BOOST YOUR IMMUNE SYSTEM: STRENGTHEN YOUR IMMUNE SYSTEM WITHOUT THE USE OF PILLS OR MEDICAL TREATMENTS

1. Camu Camu shake (6 people)

Ingredients:

- 3 spoons of camu camu powder or 1 cup of camu camu cut in cubes
- 1 cup of water
- 2 cups of chopped papaya
- 2 cups of strawberries
- 1/2 cup of ice cubes
- 2 spoons of natural honey

Procedure: In a blender mix the camu camu, strawberries and the ice. Add the honey and mix. Serve in 4 glasses. You can accompany this powerful shake with oat pancakes to make the perfect combination.

Nutritional facts: Energy 100 kcal, total fat 0 g, cholesterol 0 mg, carbohydrates 22 g and fiber 3 g.

2. Tropical shake (4 people)

Ingredients:

- 3 cups of chopped papaya
- 1 cup of chopped mango
- 1 cup of chopped strawberries
- 2 cups of natural yogurt
- 1 ½ cups of chopped pineapple
- 1 cup of ice cubes
- 2 spoons of linseed powder

Procedure: In a blender mix all the ingredients until you get a creamy look. In case you may need something to dissolve it if the juice is too dense you can add half a cup of water. Serve immediately.

Nutritional facts: Energy 194 kcal, total fat 4 g, cholesterol 7 mg, carbohydrates 35 g and fiber 5 g.

3. Beetroot delights (2 people)

Ingredients:

- 1 cup of apples cut in cubes without skin
- 1/2 cup of beetroot cut in cubes
- 4 chopped carrots without skin
- 1 cup of green tee
- 2 spoons of natural honey

Procedure: Grate the carrots, beetroot, and apples. In a blender mix the grated carrots, beetroot, apples and tee. Add honey to make it sweet. Serve in tall glasses.

Nutritional facts: Energy 252 kcal, total fat 10 g, cholesterol 8 mg, carbohydrates 44 g and fiber 5 g.

4. Energetic juice (4 people)

Ingredients:

- 1 cup of natural yogurt
- 1 banana
- 1 cup of orange juice
- 8 strawberries

Procedure: Cut the leaves off the strawberries and wash. In a blender mix all the ingredients until you get a creamy look. Serve and enjoy.

Nutritional facts: Energy 213 kcal, total fat 0 g, cholesterol 0 mg, carbohydrates 38 g and fiber 3 g.

5. Carrots extract (2 people)

Ingredients:

- 8 carrots without skin
- 2 spoons of ginger powder
- 1 spoon of linseed powder
- 1 cup of water

Procedure: Grate the carrots. In a blender mix the grated carrots, ginger, linseed and water. Add honey if needed. Serve in tall glasses. This is a great juice to have in the morning or afternoon and can be accompanied with an omelet.

Nutritional facts: Energy 221 kcal, total fat 8 g, cholesterol 11 mg, carbohydrates 64 g and fiber 5 g.

6. Vitamin C booster (3 people)

Ingredients:

- 1/2 banana
- 1/2 cup of strawberries
- 1/2 cup of orange juice
- 2 mints leafs
- 1 cup of green tee

Procedure: In a blender mix all the ingredients until you get a creamy look. In case you may need something to dissolve it if the juice is too dense you can always add a half cup of water. Serve immediately.

Nutritional facts: Energy 232 kcal, total fat 10 g, cholesterol 19 mg, carbohydrates 46 g and fiber 4 g.

7. Coconut - lemon (5 people)

Ingredients:

- 3/4 cup of lemon juice
- 4 spoons of natural honey
- 1 cup of coconut cream
- 6 ice cubes
- 1/2 cup of coconut in slices
- 1 grated lemon

Procedure: In a blender mix 1 liter of water, lemon juice, honey, coconut cream and ice. Serve and decorate with the coconut and the grated lemon.

Nutritional facts: Energy 234 kcal, total fat 9 g, cholesterol 16 mg, carbohydrates 54 g and fiber 4 g.

8. Mango delights (4 people)

Ingredients:

- 2 cups of strawberries cut in slices
- 2 bananas cut in slice
- 1 mango cut in squares
- 1 cup of natural yogurt
- 1 spoons of natural honey
- 1 cup of ice cubes

Procedure: In a blender mix the strawberries, bananas, and mango. Gradually add the yogurt until you get a creamy look. Pour a half cup to a cup of water if necessary. Add the ice cubes and mix again. Serve immediately.

Nutritional facts: Energy 256 kcal, total fat 4 g, cholesterol 8 mg, carbohydrates 68 g and fiber 4 g.

9. Oats and sesame shake (2 people)

Ingredients:

- 1 cup of almonds milk
- 1 spoon of wheat germ
- 2 spoons of toasted oats
- 1 spoon of toasted sesame seeds
- 1 spoon of almonds
- 2 spoon of natural honey

Procedure: In a blender pour the glass of almond milk; then add the wheat germ, oats, sesame seeds, and almonds. Dress with honey. Serve immediately.

Nutritional facts: Energy 259 kcal, total fat 9 g, cholesterol 14 mg, carbohydrates 32 g and fiber 7 g.

10. Quick beetroot juice (1 people)

Ingredients:

- 1 beetroot
- 1 carrot
- 1 glass of water

Procedure: Peel, cut and put the beetroot into the mixer. Cut the carrot in squares and add to the mixer. Add a glass of water and shake until you get a creamy look.

Nutritional facts: Energy 254 kcal, total fat 0 g, cholesterol 0 mg, carbohydrates 56 g and fiber 6 g.

11. Cranberry mix (1 people)

Ingredients:

- 1 cup of organic cranberry juice (250 ml)
- 1/2 cup of water
- 1 spoon of olive oil
- 2 spoons of natural honey

Procedure: Take all the ingredients and put them in the blender and mix until you get a consistent look. This a strong mix of ingredients that should be consumed early in the morning.

Nutritional facts: Energy 198 kcal, total fat 1 g, cholesterol 1 mg, carbohydrates 43 g and fiber 4 g.

12. Acid parsley juice (2 people)

Ingredients:

- 1 cup of fresh parsley
- 1 green apple
- juice of ½ lemon
- 1/2 spoon of grated ginger
- 1 cup of water

Procedure: Chop the parsley and apple. Introduce all the ingredients to the blender and mix. Strain the juice. Serve immediately. Drink before breakfast if possible.

Nutritional facts: Energy 222 kcal, total fat 4 g, cholesterol 0 mg, carbohydrates 57 g and fiber 5 g.

13. Fennel and lettuce juice (2 people)

Ingredients:

- 9 lettuce leafs (avoid the Iceberg variety which does not content so many nutrients)
- 1 slice of fresh fennel root (5 cm)
- 1 spoon of natural honey
- 1/2 cup of water

Procedure: Wash and clean the lettuce leafs and then finely chop them. Put all the ingredients in a blender and mix. Strain the juice and serve in tall glasses.

Nutritional facts: Energy 176 kcal, total fat 0 g, cholesterol 0 mg, carbohydrates 57 g and fiber 4 g.

14. Parsley shake (2 people)

Ingredients:

- 1/2 cucumber
- 100 gr of parsley
- 1/2 lactose free milk
- 1/2 cup of water
- 2 spoons of natural honey

Procedure: Wash the cucumber and parsley. Cut the cucumber in slices and chop the parsley. Put everything in the blender and mix. Strain and serve immediately.

Nutritional facts: Energy 176 kcal, total fat 6 g, cholesterol 7 mg, carbohydrates 35 g and fiber 2 g.

15. Refreshing juice (2 people)

Ingredients:

- 250 g of strawberries
- 2 pineapple slices
- 1 cup of water

Procedure: Wash the strawberries and take the green leaves out. Cut the pineapple slices in half and make sure you take the skin out. Chop the strawberries and pineapple into small pieces. Put everything in a blender and mix until you get a creamy look. Strain and when done.

Nutritional facts: Energy 189 kcal, total fat 0 g, cholesterol 0 mg, carbohydrates 22 g and fiber 2 g.

16. Grape juice (2 people)

Ingredients:

- 250 g of red grapes
- 1 cup of water
- 1/2 spoon of mint
- 2 spoons of honey

Procedure: Wash the grapes. Peel the grapes and then cut by the half to take the seeds out. Put everything in a blender and mix. Serve immediately.

Nutritional facts: Energy 165 kcal, total fat 0 g, cholesterol 0 mg, carbohydrates 36 g and fiber 4 g.

17. Good morning refresher (2 people)

Ingredients:

- 4 cups of fresh watermelon cut in cubes
- 4 spoons of lemon juice
- 1/2 cup of water
- 2 spoons of honey

Procedure: Mix everything in a blender until you get a creamy look. Dress with honey and mix again. Serve in large glasses.

Nutritional facts: Energy 175 kcal, total fat 0 g, cholesterol 0 mg, carbohydrates 28 g and fiber 3 g.

18. Radish and celery juice (2 people)

Ingredients:

- 3 cups of radishes
- 3 celery steams
- 1 cup of water

Procedure: Wash the radishes and celery. Peel the radish and cut in thin slices. Chop the celery. Add water and blend. Strain and serve immediately.

Nutritional facts: Energy 176 kcal, total fat 0 g, cholesterol 0 mg, carbohydrates 31 g and fiber 2 g.

19. Asparagus delights (2 people)

Ingredients:

- 2 asparagus
- 1 apple
- 1 broccoli steam
- 2 carrots
- 1 cup of water
- 2 spoons of natural honey

Procedure: Mix everything in a blender and add water progressively according to the consistence you want to get. Once you have a creamy look you are ready to strain the juice. Serve and enjoy.

Nutritional facts: Energy 258 kcal, total fat 3 g, cholesterol 3 mg, carbohydrates 43 g and fiber 6 g.

20. Acai-berry mix juice (2 people)

Ingredients:

- 1/2 cup of orange juice
- 1 banana cut in slices
- 1 mango cut in slices
- 1 cup of pulp of acai berries
- 1 cup of water
- 2 spoons of natural honey

Procedure: Mix everything in a blender and add water progressively according to the consistency you want to get. Once you have a creamy look serve and enjoy.

Nutritional facts: Energy 276 kcal, total fat 10 g, cholesterol 9 mg, carbohydrates 64 g and fiber 5 g.

21. Pumpkin and coco mix (2 people)

Ingredients:

- 1 glass of water
- 1 glass of coconut juice
- 1/2 cup of cooked pumpkin
- 1 spoon of honey

Procedure: In a blender mix the coconut, water and pumpkin for a few minutes until you get a creamy look. Pour the juice in tall glasses and add the honey and mix again. Enjoy.

Nutritional facts: Energy 198 kcal, total fat 2 g, cholesterol 6 mg, carbohydrates 66 g and fiber 4 g.

22. Blueberry shake (2 people)

Ingredients:

- 1/4 cup of lactose free milk
- 3/4 cup of natural yogurt
- 1 cup of blueberries
- 1 spoon of linseed powder

Procedure: Wash the blueberries. Mix everything in a blender until you get a creamy look. Add water progressively if you want a more liquid mixture. Serve immediately.

Nutritional facts: Energy 198 kcal, total fat 11 g, cholesterol 21 mg, carbohydrates 54 g and fiber 2 g.

23. Orange milkshake (2 people)

Ingredients:

- 1 cup of orange juice
- 1/2 cup of water
- 1/2 spoon of vanilla essence
- 1/2 cup of lactose free milk
- 2 spoons of honey
- 5 ice cubes

Procedure: Mix everything in a blender until you get a creamy look. Add water progressively if you want a more liquid mixture. Serve in large glasses.

Nutritional facts: Energy 212 kcal, total fat 3 g, cholesterol 6 mg, carbohydrates 48 g and fiber 2 g.

24. Popeye shake (2 people)

Ingredients:

- 1 ½ cup of green tee
- 1 cup of spinach
- 1/2 cup of water
- 1 apple
- 1 pear
- 1 spoon of honey
- 1 spoon of lime

Procedure: Wash the spinach, apple and pear. Peel the apple and pear. Chop the spinach, apple and pear. Mix everything in a blender until you get a creamy look. Add water progressively if you want a more liquid mixture. Serve and enjoy.

Nutritional facts: Energy 232 kcal, total fat 3 g, cholesterol 4 mg, carbohydrates 46 g and fiber 4 g.

25. Carrot booster (2 people)

Ingredients:

- 1 cup of pineapple cut in cubes
- 1 cup of grated carrots
- 1/2 cup of strawberries
- 1 cup of water
- juice from 2 oranges

Procedure: Mix everything in a blender until you get a creamy look. Add the water progressively if you want a more liquid mixture. Serve and enjoy.

Nutritional facts: Energy 178 kcal, total fat 6 g, cholesterol 6 mg, carbohydrates 54 g and fiber 4 g.

26. Banana-strength shake (2 people)

Ingredients:

- 3/4 cup of milk
- 1/4 cup of granola
- 1 banana
- 1 cup of ice cubes
- 2 spoons of linseed powder

Procedure: Mix everything in a blender until you get a creamy look. Add water progressively if you want a more liquid mixture. Serve immediately.

Nutritional facts: Energy 276 kcal, total fat 7 g, cholesterol 7 mg, carbohydrates 32 g and fiber 7 g.

27. Spinach mix(2 people)

Ingredients:

- 1 banana
- 1/2 cup of chopped spinach
- 1 spoon of peanut butter
- 1 ½ cup of lactose free milk
- 1 spoon of linseed powder
- 1 spoon of sesame seeds

Procedure: Mix everything in a blender until you get a creamy look. Add water progressively if you want a more liquid mixture. Serve in large glasses. Decorate with sesame seeds and enjoy.

Nutritional facts: Energy 230 kcal, total fat 9 g, cholesterol 9 mg, carbohydrates 23 g and fiber 7 g.

28. Kale power juice (2 people)

Ingredients:

- 1 cup of fresh kale
- 1 cup of almond milk
- 1 cup of blueberries
- 1/2 banana
- 1 spoon of almond butter
- 2 spoon of instant oats

Procedure: Mix everything in a blender until you get a creamy look. Add water progressively if you want a more liquid mixture. Serve immediately.

Nutritional facts: Energy 256 kcal, total fat 9 g, cholesterol 8 mg, carbohydrates 25 g and fiber 12 g.

29. Almonds and peanuts mix (2 people)

Ingredients:

- 2 cups of coconut water
- 6 almonds
- 1 spoon of vanilla essence
- 1 spoon of cinnamon
- 1 cup of chopped apple
- 1/2 cup of peanuts

Procedure: Mix everything in a blender until you get a creamy look. Add water progressively if you want a more liquid mixture. Serve in tall glasses.

Nutritional facts: Energy 218 kcal, total fat 6 g, cholesterol 5 mg, carbohydrates 46 g and fiber 4 g.

30. Blueberry booster (2 people)

Ingredients:

- 1 banana
- 1 cup of blueberries
  1/3 cup of instant oats
- 1 cup of lactose free milk

Procedure: Put the banana and blueberries in the fridge for 10 minutes. Mix everything in a blender until you get a creamy look. Add water progressively if you want a more liquid mixture. Serve immediately.

Nutritional facts: Energy 214 kcal, total fat 4 g, cholesterol 0 mg, carbohydrates 64 g and fiber 4 g.

31. Strawberry delights (2 people)

Ingredients:

- 1/2 cup of raspberries
- 1 cup of strawberries
- 1 cup of mango
- 1 cup of water
- 2 spoons of honey

Procedure: Put the fruits into the fridge for 10 minutes. Mix everything in a blender until you get a creamy look. Add water progressively if you want a more liquid mixture. Serve and enjoy.

Nutritional facts: Energy 214 kcal, total fat 5 g, cholesterol 0 mg, carbohydrates 48 g and fiber 4 g.

32. Blueberry delights (2 people)

Ingredients:

- 1 cup of raspberries
- 1 cup of blueberries
- 1 cup of strawberries
- 1/2 cup of natural yogurt
- 1/2 cup of green tee

Procedure: Mix everything in a blender until you get a creamy look. Add the water progressively if you want a more liquid mixture. Serve in tall glasses.

Nutritional facts: Energy 198 kcal, total fat 4 g, cholesterol 5 mg, carbohydrates 38 g and fiber 4 g.

33. Kiwi and strawberry mix (2 people)

Ingredients:

- 2 chopped kiwis
- 1/2 cup of chopped peaches
- 1 ½ cup of strawberries
- 1 cup of water
- 2 spoons of honey

Procedure: Mix everything in a blender until you get a creamy look. Add water progressively if you want a more liquid mixture. Serve immediately.

Nutritional facts: Energy 213 kcal, total fat 2 g, cholesterol 0 mg, carbohydrates 45 g and fiber 5 g.

34. Straw-nana juice(2 people)

Ingredients:

- 1/2 cup of chopped pineapple
- 1 banana
- 1/2 cup of mango cut in slices
- 1 cup of strawberries
- 1 cup of lactose free milk

Procedure: Mix everything in a blender until you get a creamy look. Add water progressively if you want a more liquid mixture. Serve and enjoy.

Nutritional facts: Energy 215 kcal, total fat 3 g, cholesterol 6 mg, carbohydrates 53 g and fiber 5 g.

35. Assorted delights (2 people)

Ingredients:

- 1 chopped kiwi
- 1 ½ cups of watermelon cut in cubes
- 1 ½ cups of red grapes
- 1 cup of lactose free milk
- 1 spoon of vanilla essence
- 1 spoon of honey

Procedure: Peel the grapes and then cut by the half. Take all the seeds out if they have them. Mix everything in a blender until you get a creamy look. Add water progressively if you want a more liquid texture. Serve immediately.

Nutritional facts: Energy 245 kcal, total fat 6 g, cholesterol 7 mg, carbohydrates 48 g and fiber 5 g.

36. Blue spinach (2 people)

Ingredients:

- 1 cup of blueberries
- 1 cup of peaches

  1 cup of chopped spinach
- 1/2 cup of natural yogurt
- 1/2 cup of green tee

Procedure: Put everything in a blender and mix until you get a consistent look. Add water progressively if you want a more liquid mixture. Serve in tall glasses.

Nutritional facts: Energy 238 kcal, total fat 3 g, cholesterol 7 mg, carbohydrates 54 g and fiber 5 g.

37. Strawberry smoothie (2 people)

Ingredients:

- 1/2 cup of instant oats
- 1 cup of banana
- 14 frozen strawberries
- 1 cup of lactose free milk
- 2 spoons of honey
- 1 spoon of vanilla essence

Procedure: Mix everything in a blender until you get a creamy look. Add water progressively if you want a more liquid mixture. Serve in tall glasses.

Nutritional facts: Energy 267 kcal, total fat 5 g, cholesterol 9 mg, carbohydrates 58 g and fiber 6 g.

38. Green delicate (2 people)

Ingredients:

- 1/2 cup of water
- 1 spoon of lime juice
- 2 chopped kiwis
- 1 chopped pear
- 2 spoons of honey
- 1/2 cup of ice cubes

Procedure: Mix everything in a blender until you get a creamy look. Add water progressively if you want a more liquid mixture. Serve immediately.

Nutritional facts: Energy 221 kcal, total fat 2 g, cholesterol 0 mg, carbohydrates 64 g and fiber 5 g.

39. Mango delights (2 people)

Ingredients:

- 2 mangos cut in slices
- 1 cup of natural yogurt
- 1 cup of water
- 1 banana
- 2 spoons of lemon juice
- 1 spoon of vanilla essence

Procedure: Mix everything in a blender until you get a creamy look. Add water progressively if you want a more liquid mixture. Serve and enjoy.

Nutritional facts: Energy 198 kcal, total fat 3 g, cholesterol 7 mg, carbohydrates 46 g and fiber 4 g.

40. Pineapple smoothie (2 people)

Ingredients:

- 2 cups of chopped pineapple
- 1 banana cut in cubes
- 1/2 cup of natural yogurt
- 1/2 cup of water
- 1/2 cup of ice cubes
- 2 spoons of natural honey

Procedure: Mix everything in a blender until you get a creamy look. Add water progressively if you want a more liquid mixture. Serve immediately.

Nutritional facts: Energy 236 kcal, total fat 3 g, cholesterol 7 mg, carbohydrates 58 g and fiber 6 g.

41. Cranberry smoothie (2 people)

Ingredients:

- 1 cup of natural yogurt
- 1/2 cup of cranberries
- 1 cup of bananas cut in slices
- 2 oranges cut in cubes
- 1/2 cup of water
- 3 spoons of honey

Procedure: Mix everything in a blender until you get a creamy look. Add water progressively if you want a more liquid mixture. Serve immediately.

Nutritional facts: Energy 232 kcal, total fat 3 g, cholesterol 7 mg, carbohydrates 62 g and fiber 6 g.

42. Berries mix (2 people)

Ingredients:

- 2 cups of strawberries
- 1/2 cup of blackberries
- 1/2 cup of blueberries
- 1 cup of chopped apricot
- 1 cup of water
- 3 spoons of honey

Procedure: Put all the fruits into the fridge for 10 minutes. Mix everything in a blender until you get a creamy look. Add water progressively if you want a more liquid mixture. Serve in tall glasses.

Nutritional facts: Energy 222 kcal, total fat 2 g, cholesterol 0 mg, carbohydrates 58 g and fiber 6 g.

43. Raspberry-mint juice (2 people)

Ingredients:

- 2 cups of raspberries cut in cubes
- 1 cup of water
- 1 cup of lactose free milk
- 1 cup of chopped mango
- 1/2 cup of chopped mint leafs
- 1 spoon of lemon juice
- 1 pinch of salt
- 1/2 cup of ice cubes

Procedure: Take the fruits to the fridge for 10 minutes. Mix everything in a blender until you get a creamy look. Add water progressively if you want a more liquid mixture. Serve immediately.

Nutritional facts: Energy 243 kcal, total fat 3 g, cholesterol 7 mg, carbohydrates 54 g and fiber 7 g.

44. Almond and sesame juice (2 people)

Ingredients:

- 1/2 cup of peanuts
- 1/2 cup of cherries
- 1 banana
- 1 spoon of sesame seeds
- 1 cup of almond milk
- 1 spoon of grated almonds

Procedure: Mix everything in a blender until you get a creamy look. Add water progressively if you want a more liquid mixture. Serve and enjoy.

Nutritional facts: Energy 256 kcal, total fat 5 g, cholesterol 8 mg, carbohydrates 72 g and fiber 7 g.

45. Strawberry and chia juice (2 people)

Ingredients:

- 1 spoon of chia seeds
- 1 banana
- 1 ½ cup of strawberries cut in cubes
- 1 cup of milk
- 1/2 cup of ice cubes

Procedure: Mix everything in a blender until you get a creamy look. Add water progressively if you want a more liquid mixture. Serve and enjoy.

Nutritional facts: Energy 246 kcal, total fat 3 g, cholesterol 8 mg, carbohydrates 76 g and fiber 8 g.

ADDITIONAL TITLES FROM THIS AUTHOR

70 Effective Meal Recipes to Prevent and Solve Being Overweight: Burn Fat Fast by Using Proper Dieting and Smart Nutrition

By

Joe Correa CSN

48 Acne Solving Meal Recipes: The Fast and Natural Path to Fixing Your Acne Problems in Less Than 10 Days!

By

Joe Correa CSN

41 Alzheimer's Preventing Meal Recipes: Reduce or Eliminate Your Alzheimer's Condition in 30 Days or Less!

By

Joe Correa CSN

70 Effective Breast Cancer Meal Recipes: Prevent and Fight Breast Cancer with Smart Nutrition and Powerful Foods

By

Joe Correa CSN

www.ingramcontent.com/pod-product-compliance
Lightning Source LLC
Chambersburg PA
CBHW062153020426
42334CB00020B/2587